SLEEP

SLEEP

ISHA MELLOR

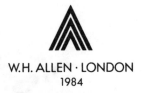

W.H. ALLEN · LONDON
1984

Typeset by Phoenix Photosetting, Chatham
Printed and bound in Great Britain
by Mackays of Chatham Ltd
for the Publishers, W.H. Allen & Co. PLC
44 Hill Street, London W1X 8LB

ISBN 0 491 02715 X

MEANING AND MYTH

O Sleep! it is a gentle thing,
Beloved from pole to pole.
To Mary Queen the praise be given!
She sent the gentle sleep from Heaven,
That slid into my soul.
                    Samuel Taylor Coleridge
                    The Rime of the Ancient Mariner

Old wives

I like to heed the sayings of these good ladies, and have looked at what they've had to say on the subject of sleep:

Beauty sleep comes before midnight.

Hear the bell and sleep well.

The best sleep in on the right side. Lying on the left causes the liver to press on the heart.

Babies must not sleep with their mothers because they can smell their milk and cry for it.

Growing children will have their vitality drawn out by old people if they sleep in the same room.

It is bad luck to sleep with a pumpkin nearby.

Sleeping with the full moon shining on the face will send you mad.

Corks in the bed will banish night cramps.

Head of the bed must point to the magnetic North.

Never, never try to wake a sleepwalker.

Phrases

Sleep like a top: When tops reach the maximum of their spin they become so steady and quiet that they are said to sleep.

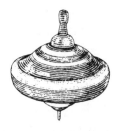

Sleepless hat: This is a worn-out and useless headgear.

Sleepers: Stout timbers on which railway lines rest; or, plain earrings to keep pierced holes open; or, spies ordered to keep a low profile in a normal life until prompted to action by their control.

Etymology

The Anglo Saxon word for sleep was *slaepen*, and the word doze is said to be a variation of the French *dors* and the Latin *dormio*. Far back in time, the word was *dermio*, which came from the Greek *derma* (a skin) because people lay on skins when they slept.

The God of sleep

The Greeks called him Hypnos, and the Romans Somnus. Child of Night and brother of Death, he lived in the underworld in a cave where the sunlight never reached. No animal life was there, and the only sound came from the River Lethe as it flowed. Poppies and other plants with soporific qualities grew near the cave. Inside, the God lay on a couch covered with sable and surrounded by empty dreams. His job was to deliver dreams as ordered by other gods to help them in their various schemings. More than once he was used to cause an awkward bout of sleep for a warrior in the Trojan war and so deviate the course of events.

Asclepius

This Greek God of Healing had many shrines and centres for healing, the most famous being at Epidaurus. Here serpents were kept for their mysterious connection with the art of cures. To this day the symbol of a snake-entwined staff is used by the medical profession.

Sufferers coming to a healing centre would go through extensive ablutions before making offerings of honey cakes. They were then led to a chamber called the *abaton* where they lay on pallets, all lights extinguished, and the silence would induce sleep. Priests kept watch and, it is believed, controlled the ensuing dreams.

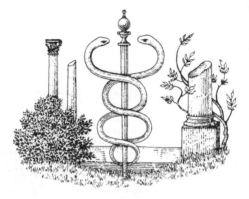

During these dreams the God Asclepius would appear with medicines and mix potions with pestle and mortar. Or he might apply a plaster to an injured limb, and even use a knife. Sometimes a snake would be made to lick the affected part. All this in dreams. The patients would wake cured, and in thankfulness later offer a votive replica in terracotta of the parts of the body that had been healed. Thus we have a vast collection of anatomical bits and bobs that can be seen in the Corinth Museum, for instance.

There are many accounts of specific cures. Blind people said that the god forced open their eyelids and poured in medicines, and they woke with sight restored. Bald men found hair beginning to sprout on their scalps after seeing the god in their dreams rubbing in ointment. If only we had the prescription today!

A woman once came to plead to become pregnant with a daughter. The god asked if she wanted anything else. No, that was all she wanted, thank you. She did conceive, and remained pregnant for three years before she felt things were not quite right. She went back to the shrine. In the second dream the god reminded her that he *had* asked if there was anything else, but she had said nothing about delivery. However, he was quite prepared to grant that also – and did! A god with a sense of humour.

The long and the short

There was a legendary and unpleasant Greek outlaw called Procrustes who lived in a region on the way to Athens. He liked to offer hospitality to travellers, insisting that they sleep on a special bed. But they had to fit it exactly. If they were too long for it they had their feet chopped off, and if they were too short he had a rack handy on which he could stretch them until they were the right length. This monster was killed by Theseus, and not before time.

Fairy tales

Sleep was used in fairy stories as an easy way of dealing with the passage of time and the effecting of transformations.

When Shakespeare tackled the realm of faery in *A Midsummer Night's Dream*, he imaginatively used this device for the scene in which Titania wakes to see Bottom wearing an ass's head and falls in love with him as if he were the handsomest of lovers.

The death curse on the Sleeping Beauty was commuted to a long sleep by the intervention of the Good Fairy. When the time was up the princess was woken by a kiss from a prince who had heard about the spell and determined to be on the spot at the right time.

The Babes in the Wood were probably saved from hypothermia when they fell asleep and the birds were able to cover them with leaves to keep out the cold.

Umbrella Man

Hans Christian Andersen wrote about a character called Ole Luk Oie who knew thousands of stories he liked to tell children. Because children are only quiet when asleep he would follow them, throw fine dust into their eyes at bedtime and blow gently on the back of their necks until their heads began to droop. Ole was a kind man, dressed in beautiful multi-coloured silks. He carried two umbrellas, one with pictures on the inside, which he spread over the good children to make them dream wonderful stories all night. Over the bad children he spread a plain umbrella that brought no dreams at all.

Tides

There is a belief that one's sleep pattern is governed by the state of the tide at the moment of one's birth. Someone born, for instance, at a 3 a.m. high tide will have a life tendency to turn night into day.

SLEEP OBSERVED

Not poppy, nor mandragora,
Nor all the drowsy syrups of the world,
Shall ever medicine thee to that sweet sleep
Which thou ow'dst yesterday.

Shakespeare
Othello

Stages of sleep

Volunteers have, for some years, been putting themselves at the disposal of scientists so that sleep and all that happens in it may be investigated. They have been wired up to instrument panels and the recorded zigzag lines have been interpreted as sleep waves.

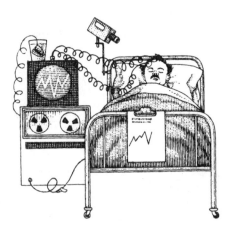

It is now known that there are four stages of slow-wave sleep. During the first two stages the sleep is light – the bodily functions slow down, muscles relax, breathing becomes shallow, and oxygen intake is reduced. The heart and pulse rates drop quite low, and the digestion process is minimal.

By the third and fourth stages, the body and nervous system are in a deeply relaxed state. During this period the restorative and repairing forces of the body are able to work. A certain chemical known as growth hormone is released, and growing children, pregnant women, those under severe mental and physical stress, and convalescents, need plenty of this.

Paradoxically, after this stage has been reached and the whole organism is at its most relaxed, it has been noted that there is a great deal of eyeball movement occurring behind the closed lids. This is called simply Rapid Eye Movement, a phrase that has slipped into our everyday vocabulary. It is during this period that we dream, and also when regenerative activity takes place in the brain cells.

During the night we repeat this cycle of four stages of slow-wave sleep divided by periods of Rapid Eye Movement (REM) four or more times in all. The REM period is about fifteen minutes, and may total about two hours.

Body clock

This is different for each person. We are larks and owls where our sleeping habits are concerned. Sometimes we have to alter this: a new job demands an earlier start to the day even though we like going to bed late and waking late. We have to be re-programmed, like computers.

This can be done gradually by going to bed half an hour earlier every day. At first, waking will occur at the same time. One will be getting less sleep, and becoming very tired. Eventually an earlier bedtime will become acceptable.

Shift workers often take many days to get used to changing from day to night work, and they sometimes feel quite ill and deprived.

A drastic method of changing our body clock is to stay awake for a full twenty-four hours and then go to bed at the new and earlier time. It may take a week or so before the body catches on to the new regime, but it will. Catnaps during the day are not allowed during such a re-training period.

Hours in sleep

Six for a man,
Seven for a woman,
Eight for a fool.
Nature requires five,
Custom takes seven,
Laziness nine,
And wickedness eleven.

There is no doubt that the boy who was never allowed to stay up late to play with the chaps in the street will grow up to be the husband who starts to yawn from half past nine onwards and try to get his wife to bed before her preferred hour of eleven. Researchers into sleeping habits say that such people are quite often sad people. They also like to get up early – and this is sad, too!

Other classifications state that people who have difficulty in getting to sleep and then wake up late are the anxious types. Those who sleep regularly from midnight to eight are dominant, sociable, and secure. Exceptionally short sleepers are angry about something.

A word of consolation for erratic sleepers with a need for plenty of catnaps: they can be as well adjusted as others with regular sleep habits, and good at dealing with crises.

Insomnia

'I never slept a wink all night.' A plea for sympathy that never gets what it asks for. It is a declaration never fully believed. I well remember my doctor saying, when I complained of insomnia, 'But you do get *some* sleep?' almost as a statement of fact. I had to admit that I did. 'So, don't worry.' I stopped worrying, and of course the bad spell began to lift.

The terrible thing about insomnia is the loneliness of the condition. As one shifts from one hot side of the bed to another, the calm breathing of a sleeping bedmate is a form of torture. It probably wouldn't disturb them if we put on the light and read, or plugged ourselves in to one of those strange all-night radio programmes. It would be better to get up and do something in another room. But we lie imprisoned in our wakefulness.

Insomniacs who live alone are more likely to leave their beds and indulge in the peculiar satisfaction of working while the rest of the world sleeps. After an hour or two they can fling themselves back between the chilly sheets and find instant sleep. This is all right if there are no neighbours to consider. Using a vacuum cleaner at 3 a.m. in a flat is bound to bring outraged complaints. I once lived in a house where the people next door had a visitor who found it hard to sleep and liked to march up and down the garden playing bagpipes. Thank goodness it was a short visit!

Occasional nights of sleeplessness will do no harm when caused by tension and difficulty in unwinding at night, but when it is obvious that a bad habit is forming, something should be done. Re-training has to be undertaken. This may take the form of following rules for relaxation, sensible eating and drinking, fresh air, exercise, and establishing a regular bedtime routine. On the other hand, the very act of entering the bedroom where nights of insomnia have been passed, can set up an association with failure to sleep. A night in a different room, even on the sofa, may sometimes do the trick.

Sleeping tablets will bring on sleep, of course, but it will not be healthy, restorative sleep. They interfere with the REM stage of sleep, those precious intervals in which emotional frustrations and problems are acted out safely.

Non-somniacs

This is a modern term for the people who experience so little sleep that it almost amounts to none at all. It is hard to imagine how they survive, but several genuine examples have been discovered in different parts of the world, and some have agreed to scientific observation to prove their claims. Such people often dispense with the routine of going to bed, and spend the night in a chair reading, or they go out to work in a second job. They keep themselves busy.

They do, however, have their periods of quiet, as well as their very short spells of sleep, which are measured in minutes rather than hours. But their records remain quite remarkable, and incomprehensible to the eight-hours-a-night brigade. How *can* non-somniacs remain healthy and normal with such lack of sleep? Do we really need a lot of sleep?

Complaining babies

Just when a mother needs to restore her strength with good sleep she may have a baby who evidently considers night to be a time for complaining. Generally she will try to pacify it with all the means suggested by clinic or hospital nurses. She will check if it is wet, too hot or too cold, or if the nappy pin is sticking into it. She will turn it onto the other side, give it a small feed or a drink of boiled water, and bring up any lurking wind. All this she will try, and still the bawling will continue. Horror stories of baby-battering pop into her mind.

Harsh advice to put the cot in another room and shut all doors between can be effective. Three nights of ignoring any cries that still penetrate have to be endured with teeth-gritting perseverance, providing the neighbours are sound sleepers.

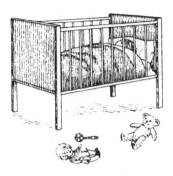

A kind grandmother coming to the rescue is the best of all cures. She will soothe the anxious mother, then carry the baby off to sleep with her for a few nights. Mother relaxes, because Grandma has been through it all and knows what to do. She sleeps blissfully, and soon feels able to cope with anything at all. Motherhood is wonderful, after all!

I was told that the reason babies cry at night is because they are hungry, and they are hungry because they are like plants and do most of their growing at night under the moon's influence. This made such sense that I was able to stop wondering if I was unwittingly poisoning my child. By the time a baby is five weeks old it usually has settled to a happy night routine of sleep – a milestone a very new mother will do well to bear in mind.

Older babies who cry at night are sometimes taken into mother's bed, thus creating a bad habit. Much better is the bright idea of dispensing with the cot and settling baby on a full-size mattress on the floor. When it cries mother can slip in with it and stay there until it falls asleep again, creeping back to her room without disturbing or re-awakening the little one.

Japanese pill

Researchers in Tokyo say they have isolated a pure and natural sleep-promoting substance obtained by crushing the brains of five thousand dead rats and injecting this into a more fortunate group of rats. These rats then sank into sleep with good and normal patterns. There are said to be no side effects.

Snoring

It is possible to get away with murder in France if it is a *crime passionelle*. Many would agree that a second exception should be the killing of a sleeping partner who snores. Nothing can be more enraging than to be woken and kept awake by the rattling and rasping in the throat of someone otherwise sleeping like a log. However one may prod or plead, the insistent noise will only be temporarily halted.

The snorer should be prevented from lying on his back, because in this position the mouth falls open and the jaw and tongue fall backward, obstructing the air passages. The air has to force its way through noisily.

Early man, always vulnerable, was particularly so when asleep, and lying on his back was worst of all because it is difficult to get up from this position. His snoring was a defence mechanism that frightened off marauding animals.

Unconsciousness

Superficially there appears to be no difference between a person in a state of unconsciousness and one who is asleep. But the former cannot be awakened until the cause of their state has worn off, whereas the latter can be roused at any time. Unconsciousness brought about by an anaesthetic or by too much alcohol is actually a form of poisoning, and until this has worn off in its own good time there is no way that arousal can be effected by outsiders shaking or shouting.

Sleep learning

Students who have to keep themselves awake during lectures by counting the number of times the speaker takes off his spectacles and puts them on again, were delighted when the new technique of sleep learning was advertised. Special tapes could be placed under the pillow to give out all the information while they slept. By morning it would all be nicely transferred to the brain, ready for later use. No more lectures, no more pouring over books. I've never met anyone who has used this method, and never heard of anyone passing exams after doing so. And now, sad to relate, scientists say these tapes simply do not do the job. It's back to the listen and read system.

Fresh thinking

Sleep is only an instinct left over from the need for animals and primitive man to get out of harm's way at night. Curled up in a safe hiding place there is no energy wasted in evading pre-dators and searching for food, and warmth is conserved. This is a survival pattern that civilised man no longer needs. However, it is so deeply embedded in his nature that he feels tired at the same time every night, whether he has been working hard or not. This shows that sleep is not required for restorative purposes. Neither is there any particular value in dreaming. Man should be freed from his compulsion to seek so many hours in sleep every night.

These theories, and others concerning sleep,

are the subject of present investigation in sleep
laboratories, and will shock all who believe firmly
that 'We are such stuff as dreams are made on.'

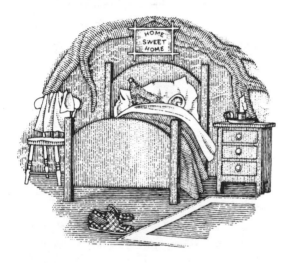

Animals

Cats and dogs have the enviable ability to fall
asleep in the best armchair and the warmest spot
in front of the fire. A pet tortoise will disappear
under a handy pile of leaves to sleep away the
frightfulness of winter, leaving us to carry on life
as best we can in the cold. Horses and cows sleep
on their feet, the cows even continuing to chew
the cud. A sloth spends twenty out of twenty-
four hours in sleep, and a bat five-sixths of its life
hanging upside down in dreamland.

Perching birds automatically lock their claws round bar or branch so that when they drop off they don't fall off! Many sea birds and swifts are believed to sleep on the wing because of the long periods they spend in flight at great altitudes. Experts do not agree on this, but I like to think there are birds up there above the clouds planing on graceful wings, eyes shut and dreaming.

Some pieces of information stick in the mind because of their strong imagery, and one such is the method of telling whether a crocodile, immobile as a tree trunk on a river bank, is really safely asleep; if all four of its legs lie pointing backwards, all you have to do is step quietly, but if they are spread out to the side, run like mad.

Sleeping creatures are vulnerable, and it is for this reason that they retire to secluded and secret places to sleep – as we disappear into our bedrooms. They will roost in high trees, burrow in holes, lairs, nests, hedges, scrub and holes in masonry. Out of sight, still and quiet, they are safe from predators. This goes for the smaller animals. Lions and bears, who have the strength and reputation of mightiness, sleep openly and long wherever they wish. An elephant, large though it may be, takes time to get going, and can easily stay awake all night if it senses that an enemy such as man or tiger lurks nearby.

READY FOR BED

But I, when I undress me
Each night, upon my knees
Will ask the Lord to bless me
With apple pie and cheese.

Eugene Field
Apple Pie and Cheese

Early to bed

Most of us have been brought up on the principle that early to bed and early to rise makes a man healthy, wealthy and wise. Doctors now say that not so much sleep as we thought is needed. Even children need not toddle off to bed as early as six o'clock – not that many do, with all the modern distractions that exist.

It is very hard for someone who feels the best part of the day starts after nine in the evening to understand why another begins to yawn then. A mother who could easily have fallen down and slept among the scattered toys on the floor at six o'clock will feel bright and alert once the evening meal is over and the house is quiet. But her spouse who came home hungry and brisk is showing al! the physical signs of sleepiness.

It really is to be wondered at that marriage survives such incompatability!

Late night drinks

Presumably, if one believes that a glass of cold water drunk just before going to bed is just the thing to promote sound sleep, then a glass of water is *de rigueur*. There can be no hard and fast rules about what to drink because we all react so differently. A surprising number of people insist on a cup of coffee, in spite of the well known fact that the caffein it contains is a stimulant. Tea is another favourite nightcap, and poor sleepers often pad along to the kitchen to brew more through the night. It is now known that tea contains even more caffein than coffee.

All milky drinks are good for sleep, because milk contains tryptophan, an amino acid which is a mild and natural sedative. Malt seems to be another aid to sleep, so we should be happy to sip those malty, chocolate-y milk drinks that conjure up images of nannies, nursery fireguards with little pyjamas warming on them, gritty tooth powder, camphorated oil – all healthy loving care. Warm milk with a spoonful of honey, itself a fine aid to sleep, is the best of nightcaps.

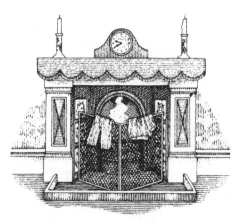

Gentlemen seem to prefer whisky, sometimes justifying their indulgence by adding hot water. Alcohol drunk late at night should be taken in small quantities, only sufficient to induce drowsiness. Too much tends to suppress the precious Rapid Eye Movement periods.

A glass of water, taken to bed in case one wakes with a dry mouth, is a kind of insurance. It is seldom needed, but if it isn't there on the bedside table one is bound to need it.

Exercise

There is no doubt that reasonable exercise during the day makes for good sleep at night. Taken last thing it is not so effective because it overstimulates the body, but of course walkies for the dog and a look at the stars make an excellent nightcap. The ideal is to have sufficient daily exercise in the open air, walking being highly recommended. Too much exertion like a sudden spurt of digging in a neglected garden will have the opposite effect because of the resulting overtiredness and aching muscles. Yoga is specifically geared to promoting sleep in natural ways by virtue of its teaching of relaxation and meditation. It must always be practised with a qualified instructor.

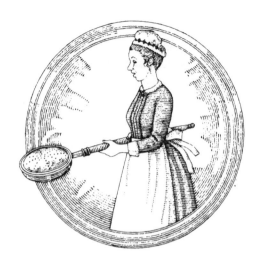

Hotties

Early bed warmers were heated bricks wrapped
in flannel. Then someone thought up the idea of
the copper warming pan. Used carefully, it was
most efficient. Embers of fires in the hearth were
loaded into the pan, the lid fastened down, and
the whole thing slipped between the sheets and
directed across and down into every chilly spot of
the bed. Naturally, if this was done by a servant,
all the master and mistress had to do was jump in
while all was cosy. Doing it oneself after undres-
sing in a cold bedroom would have been another
matter. And if a hot coal escaped and burnt holes
in the precious sheets, that was very bad news.

The disappearance of coal fires gave us an old-world decoration to hang on our walls and yet another bit of copper to polish.

Stone hot water bottles of a horrible putty colour were fine to start the night with, but shocking toe-stubbers later on – and it was inadvisable to kick them out of bed when no longer needed.

Rubber hot water bottles are much more endearing, and simply ask to be cuddled. I do however dislike the way they glug at me through the night!

The electric blanket was a welcome invention, either under or over the body, but there is often a lingering fear that the electricity will go wrong and turn us into burnt toast. The advent of the duvet with its all-enveloping warmth has diminished the need for electric blankets.

Dozens of everything

Up to the start of this century it was quite usual for a bride's trousseau to contain two or three dozen nightdresses. As these were voluminous and trimmed with much lace and embroidery, it must have taken years to produce this part of the wardrobe alone. And how sick she must have grown of them all before they wore out!

Man under the bed

It is an old joke that spinsters always look hopefully under the bed for a man. But it is children who suffer real terror at bedtime. Not so very long ago most bedrooms were only lit by candles. There was no click of a switch to illuminate the room before crossing the threshold. The flickering candle flame cast horrifying shadows on the walls, and the space under the bed was occupied in childish imaginations by robbers, murderers, creepies, and slimies – all waiting to attack.

Robert Louis Stevenson knew just how children felt when he wrote:

> Must we to bed indeed? Well then,
> Let us arise and go like men,
> And face with an undaunted tread
> The long black passage up to bed.

Royal nightgowns

Anne Boleyn had what must have been a very seductive nightgown of black satin bordered with black taffeta and velvet, which sounds more like a ballgown to us today. The queens of France had to obey very strict rules of mourning, and these extended to the wearing of black in bed for six weeks.

Queen Elizabeth went in for nightwear almost as sumptuous as her day wear. She had one nightgown that was lined with fur and decorated with gold lace, a mixture of cosiness and scratchiness. A more simple number, worn on summer nights perhaps, was of cambric 'wrought' all over with black silk. Yet another took twelve yards of purple velvet 'frized' with white and russet silk.

Henry Tanworth Wells painted the famous picture of the young Victoria roused from bed and still in her nightdress receiving from Ministers the news that she was now Queen of England.

Pyjamas

Pyjamas for women were first introduced in the 1890s and called the Combination Night Gown. They took four and a half yards of calico or flannel. For men, Dr Jaeger made a pure wool night suit and with it went a natty wool helmet buttoning under the chin. Striped pyjamas, which are still the most popular ones, first appeared in Peter Robinson's 1902 catalogue.

Practical and instantly comfortable garments they may be, but they do tend to become restricting and over-warm as night progresses. Handkerchiefs stuffed into their breast pockets often form lumps that work round under the ribs. Men of the older generations still bemoan the disappearance of the woven pyjama cord, even though its unthreading created major crises from time to time in the mad search for a bodkin and a practical woman to effect the re-thread.

Masks

How unreasonable it seems that we can fall asleep in a chair in full daylight but must have complete darkness in our bedrooms at night. Lined curtains and blinds are expensive and keep out fresh air. A black sleep mask, softly padded and comfortably fastened is a cheap solution. In the first class area of an airliner they are issued free to passengers, but as an ordinary tourist I make do with a black sock or dark scarf.

Windows

The two categories of sleepers: those who like the windows open whatever the weather, and those who want them tightly shut except perhaps in high summer, can never be reconciled. It is no use trying.

Top gear

Nightcaps used to be essential items of night-wear. Those worn by women seem to have been like mob caps, and ordinary men went in for those long pointed ones with a tassel at the apex. But there was a time when they were elaborate and precious enough to be bequeathed in Wills, being made of velvet and decorated with gold thread. They carried a health hazard, it seems, for there was a warning that there should be a hole in the top for the purpose of ventilation and the preservation of the teeth!

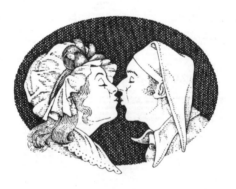

Simple nightcaps are coming back into fashion, and doctors agree that old people should certainly wear them to stave off the danger of hypothermia, since up to eighty per cent of body heat is esti-mated to be lost through the top of the head.

BEDS AND COVERS

Matthew, Mark, Luke and John,
The bed be blest that I lie on.
Thomas Ady
A Candle in the Dark

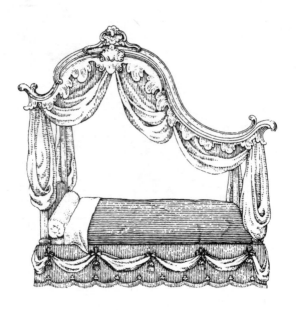

Beds of the past

The word 'bed' originally referred to the materials upon which one slept, such as skins. Only since the sixteenth century has it come to include the actual bedstead.

Ancient Egyptian beds must have been very uncomfortable, from what one may observe in museums. They were of solid wood, with no mesh of any kind, and sloped upwards to the head, where a wooden neck rest was placed.

In Tudor and Stuart times the bed was the most important article in the house; and we've all heard of Shakespeare's Second Best Bed which he so generously left to Anne Hathaway in his Will.

The term fourposter could appear to be a misnomer from the fact that the head posts were concealed by the curtains and only the foot posts left exposed. The curtains hung from the tester or roof of the bed, and were drawn right round at night to keep out draughts, and for privacy.

At the end of the eighteenth century beds were more simple, with short head and foot boards and prettily turned short posts. They had no tester or all-round curtains.

An early eighteenth century terrace house often had a cupboard bed on the top landing. Here a wretched serving maid would have to undress before climbing onto a mattress-topped chest in which she had to keep all her belongings. Then she would shut the cupboard doors that enclosed the chest, and lie there out of sight. The cupboard had no roof to it – a generous arrangement enabling her to breathe.

A most elegant bed known as a Sleigh or French Bedstead was much favoured in the United States in the 1850's. It was low, with curved and scrolled matching head and foot. It was the sort of bed or couch on which fairy princesses languished while waiting for the prince to arrive.

Today's beds

Victorian brass beds are very popular at present, and there must be a factory somewhere which reproduces the hollow bedknobs that had a habit of working loose and getting lost. My grandmother's beds were wonderful iron framed ones with black rails and brass finials that rattled and clinked every time one turned over.

Wooden beds offered scope for carving on head and foot boards. Then suddenly they were out of fashion – the divan had arrived. Later still this was called the studio couch, which meant that it was pushed up against a wall and smothered with day cushions.

Camp beds used to be made of canvas attached to wooden trellis sides that scissored up for storage. Now one simply blows up an air bed.

A modern home will probably have a king-size bed in the main bedroom and singles in other ones. The large beds may be rectangular, oval or round. The headboard can have a complicated control panel for opening doors throughout the house, drawing curtains, switching on radio and television, setting up soothing rocking motions, playing back the answering machine, organising alarm calls and making drinks.

Togetherness

The best example of this is the Great Bed of Ware, said variously to accommodate twenty couples, twenty-six butchers and their wives, or a troop of soldiers. But this rhyme sounds more realistic:

At Ware was a bed of dimensions so wide
Four couples might cosily lie side by side,
And thus without touching each other abide.

Its style and workmanship date it from the time of Elizabeth I. It measured overall ten feet seven inches in width, ten feet ten inches in length; and it stood eight feet nine inches high. The mattress was nine feet square. It received its name from the town of Ware in Hertfordshire where it was housed in various inns for a good two hundred years, after probably having started life in Ware Manor, once the property of the Earls of Huntingdon.

Both Shakespeare in *Twelfth Night* and Ben Jonson in *The Silent Woman* make reference to the bed. It has passed through the hands of many antiquarians, and Charles Dickens tried to buy it for a hundred pounds. It now stands in the Victoria and Albert Museum where one may look and wonder about the reputation of haunting, of 'pinching, nipping and scratching' experienced by its occupants. Were they due to ghostly or more solid presences?

Primitive men and women slept in groups with feet pointing towards the fire. This was an efficient form of togetherness that gave protection from sudden attack.

The old habit of mothers having their babies in bed with them had to be discouraged because of the terrible number of baby deaths caused by Mama turning over carelessly in the night.

Some users of double beds complain about 'half the bed and all the clothes', but well adjusted sleeping partners enjoy the comfort of sharing and are very unhappy when made to sleep apart.

Rock-a-bye baby

When Moses was parked in the bullrushes it was in the most basic of cradles, a woven basket; but his name has been given to all such portable beds ever since. Poor Jesus had to make do with a wooden manger, and though the fashion has not stuck, it highlights a poignant story.

Old paintings of domestic interiors frequently depict the solid wooden cradle on rockers set near the mother's chair so she can keep it rocking with her foot while her hands are busy with peeling vegetables or sewing. Very Important Babies sometimes slept in miniature fourposters mounted on rockers, and there was a clever space-saver called a truckle bed that was stowed under the big bed during the day and trundled out for an older child at night.

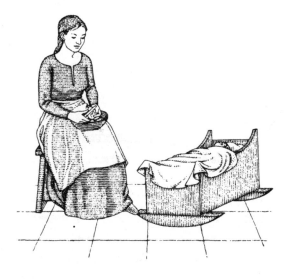

The prettiest cradles were those that swung from iron frames. They were lined and covered with removable fabrics, often in two or three layers of lawn, organdie and lace. A tall bent arm was fixed at the head and over this curtains were draped to fall in a graceful vee to keep draughts away. This arm always ended in a shepherd's crook to which could be tied the appropriate bow of pink or blue, and from which was suspended a porcelain angel or cherub to guard the new soul.

The modern carry-cot borrows the best from all these examples. Portable as the Moses basket, padded and lined as wanted, able to be set in a folding frame in the nursery, direct into the pram for an outing, or on the back seat of the car – all without disturbing that creature we are so scared of, a sleeping baby.

Bed making

Great featherbeds of the past needed more than one person to make them daily. The method was to take hold of each corner and shake the feathers into a central mound. This then had to be evenly distributed by beating with a bedstick or bed-staff. A lollipop-shaped gadget called a bed smoother was used to impart a finishing touch.

An American statistic once officially stated that a housewife walked the equivalent of four miles and spent twenty-five hours a year in making a double bed daily. Young people mostly eschew all bedmaking, and even manage to make a bed furnished with a duvet look unmade!

Hospital patients soon learn that there is one way and one way only of making a bed. Envelope corners have to be mastered as soon as they can totter out. But a hospital bed is not a cosy place in which to lie. Covers are tucked in so tightly that toes have to remain *en pointe*, and the tops are turned back so far they stop at the waist and let in all the draughts.

In many Continental countries the bedroom windows in the morning will have duvets billowing out of them to freshen and to fluff up the down. In Britain there used to be strict rules about stripping beds. All the covers were taken off and hung over chairs to air and the mattress humped double and left for at least two hours before the bed was re-made. In chilly damp bedrooms this was an invitation to rheumatism.

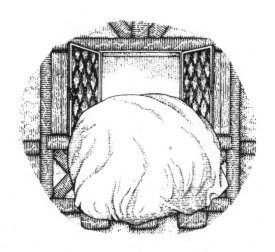

Shopping

When buying a new bed always lie on it in the shop. No need to take off your shoes, since the salesman will provide a little mat for your feet to rest on. You should, however, remove your coat so that you can relax better. But the chances are that you will feel terribly embarrassed by sly glances from passing customers, and you'll jump up again almost at once, pronouncing the bed very comfortable. There is only one person whose judgment I would like to have when I buy a bed – the princess who was so sensitive she was able to feel a pea under twelve mattresses. She'd know what was what.

Apple pie bed

Never were my stitches so close or even as when sewing up the ends of pyjama legs for an unfortunate victim. A few choice holly leaves were sometimes inserted as a finishing touch.

But the traditional method of making an apple pie bed is to remove the top sheet and fold it in half crossways. Then it is placed back on the bed, the lower half just beneath the pillow, and the top half turned back in the usual way over the blankets. The innocent occupant will jump in, stretch the legs towards the bottom of the bed, and come up hard against the fold. The bed then has to be remade, and the resulting fury will very likely banish all inclination for sleep. Worst of all, if the sheet is well-worn the feet may have gone right through.

Other embellishments may be the sprinkling of pepper on the pillow, hairbrushes at the end of the bed, squeakers under the bottom sheet. There is no end to the tricks an inventive and malicious mind can think up. It is of course imperative for the perpetrators to listen outside the door for the howls of anguish.

Mattresses

The first mattresses were filled with straw or hay and called palliasses, from the French for straw. Then the word pallett came to mean a small and roughly made bed. Such mattresses must have provided homes for livestock just waiting for an orgy of human blood-sucking as well as being very prickly. The phrase 'hitting the hay' comes from the time when we slept on such mattresses.

A cheap filling was flock that was carded wool refuse or shoddy (shredded old cloth). Its only advantage was that it was slow to burn, for it flattened quickly and produced a hard and lumpy surface to lie on.

Feather mattresses that mounded up all round the body were a distinct improvement, but hot in summer and requiring all that daily shaking up.

Wool comes and goes in fashion as a filling, but it needs re-making regularly. In parts of France itinerant workers toured from house to house in summer to desembowel the family mattresses, card the wool into high mountains of fluff, and stuff it back into the washed covers or into new ones. Then they stitched with great needles, anchoring through rosettes of wool and making the whole resemble the buttoning of a Chesterfield. This work was carried out on the spot, preferably in the sunshine of the garden, so a watch could be kept on every last shred of fibre and no filching could take place. Suspicious maybe, but sensible.

Horsehair could be mixed with the wool, but it tended to break down the wool into dust more quickly, and to work through and prickle sleepers. Stern Victorians favoured mattresses made entirely of horsehair.

Latex foam, which is made of rubber, has many admirers. It also comes in varying degrees of firmness, and a mattress made of this needs only occasional turning. It has a long life, provided the bedroom is not overheated. Its non-admirers are warm-blooded people who say that it does not allow the body to breathe sufficiently. To be on the safe side, I would avoid every other kind of foam in case it turns out to be the type that in a fire produces deadly fumes that kill in just thirty seconds.

A good modern sprung mattress is costly. Pocketed springs that compress independently of neighbouring springs provide the answer for heavy husbands and lightweight wives who would otherwise roll towards the middle of the bed. One half of the bed can be firmer than the other for partners with differing requirements, and there are double beds that can be unzipped down the middle to make two single ones for the odd occasion when togetherness isn't all it's cracked up to be.

Orthopaedic mattresses are specially hard sprung ones and designed for back sufferers. But because one cannot please everybody, there are those who say that they *give* them backache.

The invention of the water bed for home use has been the source of many funny jokes, but those who can afford them say they are absolute bliss. Hospitals have long employed them for patients with certain injuries that cannot bear pressure.

Whatever one's mattress, it is certain that when one begins to wake in the morning feeling more tired than when one went to bed, it is time to think about a visit to the nearest bedding centre.

Duvets

'An end to bed making', the advertisers claimed. And eventually the British public responded and went in for the *doovay*, only to discover undreamt of complications.

A bed furnished with a duvet leaves a lot exposed. It doesn't reach to the floor, so something has to be done about the space underneath where suitcases lurk amid the fluff. A valance has to be bought to fill in this gap, a valance that has to match the undersheet that matches the pillow cases that match the removable duvet cover. Quite a massive co-ordination exercise. Then changing the duvet cover is like trying to stuff a giant ballon into a paper bag, and before one can get the various corners aligned one has almost had to crawl inside. All very exhausting, and not at all what the advertisers had promised.

DROPPING OFF

O ye who are about to sleep, commend your souls
to Him who never sleeps.

> From *The Sacred Books of Buddha*

Courting sleep

Who first thought of counting sheep as a way of getting off to sleep? Was it really a shepherd who found himself nodding as he counted his flock into the pen then tried it out when he got home to bed? We are apt to find that sleep escapes us the more we dwell on our day's work.

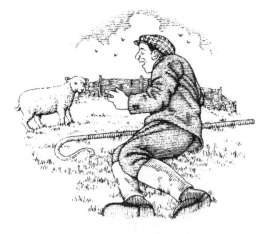

Children play counting and word games when they go to bed to keep themselves awake rather than to invite sleep, though sleep soon gets the better of them before they get anywhere near a hundred or Z. Grown-ups will try to remember poems they once knew by heart, make up speeches for various occasions, compose menus, and end up worrying too much and chasing sleep away.

I have two methods which work for me. One is to get out of bed and wander about until I feel chilly. Then the relief of snuggling back under the sheets is so comforting that sleep takes over at once. The other is to go through the acts of the day, but in precise reverse. I start with the moment of stretching out in bed, before that, of getting into bed, of putting on my nightdress. Then, when did I actually turn out the light? After lying down, or before? Start again. This time I may get back as far as the moment I set out to go to the library, and then I find I can't remember what time it was when I spoke to my sister on the telephone. Although I've recommended this exercise to many people, I've never heard of anyone reaching as far back as breakfast. Sleep becomes a blessed escape.

Lullaby

To study a lullaby is to understand how onomatopoeic or echoic it is in nature. The words have a hushing sound that soothes. The word s-l-e-e-p is repeated over and over, and mingled with some lulla-lulla's and hushabye's. The accompanying music has a rocking rhythm, and it isn't long before baby gets the message and drifts into the beautiful land of nod.

Some of the tricks

Lay a hand on your heart and concentrate on its beats.

Imagine yourself in a room lined entirely with black velvet.

Plan the spending of a fortune.

Experience the sensation of seeing through the third eye, which is supposed to be situated above the bridge of the nose.

Listen to the ticking of the clock.

Feel yourself walking towards a huge white sheet.

Pretend that you have got to get up.

Relax every part of the body in sequence, from the toes up.

Repeat the word 'sleep' over and over again.

Think of waves breaking on the shore.

Yawn.

Try to recall the names of all the teachers at your school.

Plan a herbaceous border.

Try to stay awake.

Catnaps

There is a feeling of guilt about catnapping. We hate ourselves for falling asleep while listening to a radio play only to wake as the announcer reads the cast list. Now we'll never know if it was the lover or the butler. Day sleep is a perverse phenomenon. The moment someone says, 'Just put your head back and have a nice nap,' we become instantly wide awake. Catnapping is escapism, and one cannot escape if someone is watching.

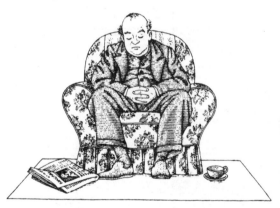

It may help to know that the habit is said to belong to well-adjusted humans, and that leaders of nations indulge in it because they spend the night guarding our interests. The medical term for uncontrollable attacks of day sleep is narcolepsy, which is no help at all.

Herbs

Balm, chamomile, elder flower, hyssop, lime flower, marigold, melilot, peppermint, poppy, rue, valerian, and vervain are leading names among plants for inducing sleep. And what beautiful names they are. Most of them can be made into tisanes for late night drinks. Peppermint essence in a little hot water is particularly effective in this way, and also lettuce leaves boiled for a few minutes in water. Chamomile and lime flowers can also be added to baths at night for a soothing effect. While considering how plants help us in our quest for sleep, it is very strange to discover that the green coffee bean is used in homeopathic potency to make a sleep medicine.

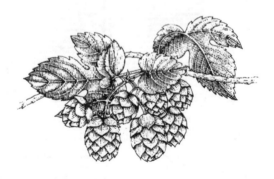

Hop pillows

These are prominent in gift shops and promise peaceful nights. Sceptics say it is only a matter of auto-suggestion, but they should consider the fact that people are often overcome with drowsiness if they enter an oast house in operation. George III is said to have been very keen on using such pillows. If the scent of hops is not entirely liked, pillows with the addition of other fragrant herbs are to be found. A word of advice: all herb pillows should have their fillings changed every three months.

Legs

'Got the fidgets in my legs. Can't get to sleep.' This state is distressing and uncontrollable, and has so baffled medics investigating the problem of insomnia that they haven't been able to stick a Latin tag on it. They simply refer to it as Restless Leg Syndrome.

Sex

Happy are those who can experience satisfying sexual intercourse at night and so benefit from the deep and natural sleep that follows it. This happy result must be why the term 'sleeping with' is used by those who certainly do not go to bed primarily for sleep.

Loving memory

'What are you writing about next?' a dear friend asked me. 'Sleep' I told her, and asked if she had any good advice about ways of getting off to sleep. 'Oh, yes. But wait a minute. I'll just make sure my old man's not listening.' Back she came to the telephone and spoke in a hushed voice: 'Counting my past lovers – trying to remember their names.' 'How many?' I asked. 'Twenty-one so far.' Could that really send her off to sleep, I wondered?

Heartbeat

A clever device for inducing sleep in babies is a recording of a woman's heart beating. It takes baby back to the time in the womb when it was enveloped in this comforting rhythmic sound. It also works well with puppies.

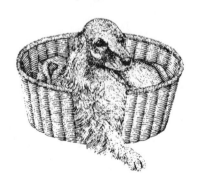

DREAMS

For you dream you are crossing the Channel, and
tossing about in a steamer from Harwich –
Which is something between a large bathing
machine and a very small second class carriage.

> Sir William Schwenck Gilbert
> *Iolanthe*

An A B C of dreams

Apple	Generally a good omen. If sweet, well earned rewards – sour, loss.
Book	Slow, steady progress. Pleasant life ahead.
Chair	An empty chair means unexpected news, sitting in a cosy one foretells comfort, and a rocker possible inheritance.
Disaster	A dream of the opposite.
Envelope	An obstacle.
Fire	An appeal for help from a close person.
Grass	Mowing it means sad news, and sowing it future security but not luxury.
Hospital	A hospital visit indicates surprising news.
Insult	A contrary dream. Loyalty from friends.
Jam	Happy domesticity.
Kitten	Romance for a woman, disappointment in love for a man.
Loss	A contrary dream.
Mint	Happiness.

Newspaper	If reading it, distant events will be in one's favour.
Orchids	Extravagance should be curbed.
Poetry	Writing it means a new friend will be made.
Quarrel	With a stranger this means change of residence.
Rats	Trouble through jealousy.
Snow	To shovel it means help is coming from friends.
Telephone	Warning of unexpected rivalry. If out of order sad news is on the way.
Umbrella	Security, unless broken or torn – then delays.
Vomit	Financial improvement for the poor and the opposite for the rich.
Whip	Used on an animal, an injustice is on your mind. Make amends.
X-ray	Good health.
Yell	To yell is good news. If others yell it is bad news.
Zip	A stuck zip equals a social disaster.

Recall

'I had such an amazing dream last night . . .' And there it stops. The harder the dreamer tries to remember, the more hazy the memory becomes. A certain equatorial race had good advice on the subject: 'If you have a strange dream, rise at once and ponder over it.' Ancient Egyptians training to become priests had to keep a wax tablet next to their beds so they could record their dreams with a special stylus as soon as they woke. Before settling to sleep the next night they would erase these recordings with a roller – an action symbolising a clearing of the mind to receive fresh instruction from the spirit world in dreams.

Modern investigators have found that it is the rational people who have the best recall, and the intuitive who have the most difficulty. To help in retaining memory of dreams one should try to withdraw gradually from their realm and cross slowly from night to day, with no sudden shock of awakening.

Premenstrual tension

Medical investigation has found that the dreams of women suffering such tension are often of a most violent nature, and such violence is frequently directed against loved ones.

A prophetic dream

Abraham Lincoln had such a dream only one week before his assassination. He dreamt that he left his bed and wandered through the rooms of the White House, coming upon some soldiers standing guard round a catafalque on which lay a corpse. People were standing around weeping, but the face of the corpse was covered and he couldn't see who it was. 'Who is dead?' he asked. 'The President – killed by an assassin.' Lincoln coolly recorded that he slept no more that night and was strangely annoyed by the dream thereafter.

Inspiration

Writers, composers and mathematicians sometimes go to bed with creative problems unsolved, and wake in the morning with solutions ready and clear in their minds. While they slept inspiration went to work.

The poet Coleridge fell asleep one afternoon in his Devon cottage after he'd been reading about Khan Kubla and his palace. When he woke he knew he had composed in his sleep hundreds of lines on the subject, and he sat down to write before he forgot it all. The words flowed easily, and then there was a knock at the door. A man with a message from nearby Porlock detained him for a while. Admirers of the poet refer with hate to this Person From Porlock, because on returning to his writing Coleridge could not recall another word. We are left with but a fragment of what we should have had, the fifty-four lines that begin, 'In Xanadu did Kubla Khan a stately pleasure-dome decree,' and end 'For he on honey-dew hath fed, And drunk the milk of Paradise.'

Artistic nightmares

The artist Fusili painted horrific pictures, and would eat raw beef and pork chops last thing at night to make sure he would suffer nightmares to provide him with rich subject matter.

Physical jerks

The very physical sensation of falling down stairs so that the legs give a great jerk are much more connected with the process of letting go into sleep than with dreaming. Drawing the feet up in terror as the gigantic spider approaches at the end of the bed is the same kind of thing. This theory makes sense when one realises that these jerks happen very soon after one has relaxed in bed. The medical term is Nocturnal Myoclonus.

Dream therapy

We have all heard of Dr Freud's theories concerning the symbolism of dreams. As a result we are often hesitant to recount our dreams because of the sexual connotations we unwittingly reveal in so doing. The most innocent objects like cigars, guns, chair legs and umbrellas may be classed as phallic symbols, putting an interpretation on the dream that may be nothing like the adventure we remember. However, there are practitioners classed as dream therapists, trained psychiatrists who have been able to treat physical and mental disorders by study and interpretation of a sufferer's recurrent dreams.

The wandering spirit

Heraclitus said that 'to those who are awake there is one world in common, but to those who are asleep each is withdrawn into a private world of his own.'

Dreams of swimming or crawling through small spaces are images of the spirit returning to the body.

The odd thing about sleepwalking is that it does not happen while one is actually dreaming. It is usually an inherited habit, and practised mainly by males.

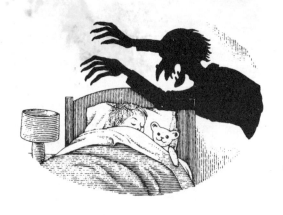

Nightmares

When I began to do research for this book, I asked many people to tell me about their nightmares. The strange thing was that they so often said, 'I don't really have them,' and then went on to describe the most horrifying dream. Some shuddered and pretended not to remember.

Many nightmares are concerned with escape and chase. We run with ever weakening legs from monsters, are menaced by machinery, and try to catch trains as they gather speed. One of the great reliefs of life is waking up safe in our beds just before we are pushed into the threshing machine or gobbled up by the giant snake with the head of our old headmistress.

My brother, who always sleeps lying on his stomach, had for a time to lie on his back because of a neck injury. During this time he had an understandable but really nasty dream. He lay on a bed made entirely of cotton wool in which were embedded hundreds of razor blades on edge. Terror of being cut into spaghetti made him sweat with the effort of trying to levitate.

The nightmare of my early childhood would occur when spending the night at my Grandmother's house, and must have been the result of too many chocolate eclairs. An airship would come in through the bedroom window and bite me in the stomach with its pointed end. However much it was pointed out that there was a slight difference between the size of the window and the airship, I would howl, 'But it did, it did – and it hurt!'

Later I had another recurring nightmare that sometimes contained a cruel inversion. I would dream that an arm or a leg had been amputated, and I was trying to face the world with this shocking loss. Most of all I dreaded the pity and disgust of my school friends. I knew exactly how it would feel, the irrevocable disaster that no one in the world could repair. Waking brought the big test. How reluctantly did my right hand feel for the left arm or the right foot for the left. (It was curiously always a left limb that had been lost.) Oh, what a relief when it finally sank in that it had all been a dream! The cruel inversion? Dreaming that I had woken up and found it to be a dream, and now being really awake. Where was the truth? And in those days there wasn't the comfort of micro-surgery.

Future husband

Unmarried girls should sleep with a piece of wedding cake under the pillow. This will bring a dream of a future husband.

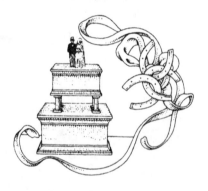

SLEEPING OUT

Old Meg she was a Gipsy,
And she liv'd upon the Moors:
Her bed it was the brown heath turf,
And her house was out of doors.

John Keats
Meg Merrilies

Straws in the wind

A delightful citizen of the world with a great store of human stories and a readiness to relate them over a cup of lemon tea, told me the following tale of a gentleman of the road.

During my friend's last year at school he had the common disagreement with his parents about the time he was coming home at night. One night he found himself locked out. He could find no convenient window to force open. It was winter and there had been a little early snow. He wandered to the park and tried to settle on one of the few empty benches. Strange mounds occupied most of them – the tramps and winos of the day. His overcoat soon became inadequate to keep out the cold, and he was just about to get up when he was approached by one of the tramps.

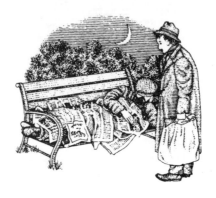

'Here, let me make you a proper bed,' the man said, taking out from inside his layers of garments several newspapers. He laid some neatly on the bench and told the lad to lie down again. Then he covered him in such a way that he was in a cocoon of newsprint. Finally, he handed him two drinking straws printed with the name of a famous cafe. 'You'll need these.' 'What for?' 'Put one in each nostril, then if the snow falls heavily and you get buried while you sleep you'll have two air holes.'

The spoken word

I feel so sorry for the lecturer when a member of the audience falls asleep and starts to snore. So I always try to stop the noise before the speaker becomes aware of it. If the snorer is sitting in front of me I sometimes give the chair a little kick, but this can result in a startling arousal. What is needed is a method of getting through to the sleeper so that he will wake naturally, not knowing that he has been deliberately disturbed. I've found that a short sharp sound like snapping the clasp of a handbag or letting the heel of my shoe drop against the floor – sounds quite natural in a hall of listeners – does the trick beautifully, even with someone sitting at a distance from me.

Up comes the head, slowly, shoulders square discreetly, eyes fix in concentration on the platform. There is no feeling of guilt because the subject believes he has drifted off and back with no one the wiser.

Motorway

I used to enjoy dozing in the car while my husband drove, particularly in motorway scenery. But not any more. Once, driving alone up the M1, he began to feel drowsy, noted that a service station was only another ten miles off, and pressed on. The next thing he knew the car was entangled in the fencing on the central reservation. He was unhurt, thank goodness, but now he heeds the early warning. And when I'm his passenger I stay awake and chat.

The cold shoulder

Oh, the public shame of the situation! In a train the man next to me falls asleep. His head droops sideways and lands on my shoulder. However I twitch and squirm it stays put, with the threat of sliding down to my bosom. Travellers sitting opposite look the other way or hide behind their newspapers. What can I do? The man will feel so awful when he wakes, and when he apologises I'll have to say, 'It's all right, really,' as if I enjoyed being taken for a PLP (Public Leaning Post). The only solution costs money. It is to slip neatly from under the human burden and spend the rest of the trip in the buffet car.

Boarding school

How many times have we wept as we read of a miserable little new boy crying his heart out in homesickness under the rough sheets and thin blankets on his first night in the dorm? Our consolation lies in the knowledge that the book would not have been written if there were not to be a happy ending with the boy developing into the hero of the Upper Fifth – but on that first night he doesn't know this, poor fellow.

I remember a description of a much despised boy who invented a wonderful self-fuelling method of keeping his feet warm in bed. He got a length of rubber tubing as long as himself and put one end near his feet and the other in his mouth. The flow of warm air did the trick most efficiently, but his schoolmates said his feet would soon drop off after being exposed to such an overdose of his bad breath.

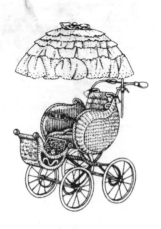

Sleep on wheels

Our first experience of this comes when we are wheeled in prams, and a liking for it can remain for the rest of our lives. It left generations with a desire to hop onto the Orient Express, Blue Train, Transiberian Express, Golden Arrow, Coromandel Express, Royal Scot, and Canadian Pacific – but a few of the world's wonderful trains.

Travellers in sleeping cars doze fitfully through the night, waking at ghostly stations echoing with shoutings, spittings, and clankings. They try not to think about shivering in their pyjamas by the side of the track if there should be a derailment. Then suddenly it's morning, and hot coffee is available, with crusty rolls that take the skin off the roof of the mouth. Sleeping on a train is wonderful!

Return to civilisation

It can be a problem for explorers when they return from the wilder regions of the world to adjust to the comforts of the bedroom. They simply cannot get to sleep in a good bed. Bearers of morning cups of tea have often stumbled over a blanketed body lying on the floor. Such travellers can take a long time to get out of the habit of sleeping rough.

Snakes

When travelling in snake-infested country and having to sleep on the ground, a wise precaution is to arrange a rough and hairy rope around the space on which it is proposed to spend the night. Snakes hate crossing anything that prickles their undersides, and so will not follow up any desire to snuggle down with a human. If no sufficiently hairy rope is handy a smooth one can be studded with thorny twigs and prickly leaves.

Sleep, baby, sleep

My first son, usually easy to settle for the night, refused to do so when staying away from home, even at Grandma's. No sooner would I settle downstairs for gossip and sherry than his pyjama'd form would sidle round the door and report, 'Mummy, there's a dragon on top of the wardrobe.' So at last I decided, after a battle of wills, to stay with him in the first place until he fell asleep. What happened? I fell asleep across the foot of the bed and had to be woken before the macaroni cheese was taken out of the oven. The second son gave no trouble in this way, but then he had his brother to talk to in bed. Their young sister's behaviour was a mixture of the two. Sometimes she settled happily and sometimes she saw eagles or thought the house was on fire. One has to be prepared for anything if one is a mother.

WAKING UP

Awake! for Morning in the Bowl of Night
Has flung the Stone that puts the Stars to Flight.

Edward Fitzgerald
Omar Kayyam

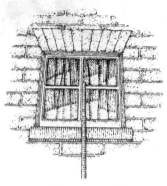

Alarm calls

These are hated by everyone. In the past it was possible to direct this hatred against a particular person – the knocker-up who banged with a long pole on bedroom windows to rouse miners and mill workers for the early shifts. Now we hurl abuse at the alarm clock. Very heavy sleepers find it difficult to get one loud enough to do the job. They make do with what they've got by placing it in a metal bowl with a handful of coins to aug-

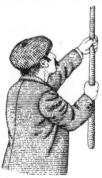

ment the noise – which is but one of the ingenious adaptations. There is always the danger of waking up when the alarm first blasts, shutting it up and falling asleep again. So it is quite a good idea to place the clock on the other side of the bedroom so one has to get out of bed to silence it. Telephone alarm calls are reliable and cannot be ignored. Variation comes in the tone of the operator's voice which may be apologetic, impersonal, or almost gloating.

Banging the head on the pillow before going to sleep, seven times for a seven o'clock waking, for instance, works for people with plenty of confidence, but is quite hopeless for those who cannot even trust alarm clocks to go off on time, and keep waking through the night to check.

Where were we?

Sometimes when we wake it is as if we've been very busy all night. There is a sense of having been on a journey. But where have we been? All we have to go on are memories of dreams. We may feel that there have been spiritual experiences during our wanderings through the continent of sleep. Perhaps our dreams are ley lines to something beyond.

Animal calls

The traditional morning call from the animal world is the cock, and various domestic animals have their special ways of rousing their owners. My father's ginger cat used to sit on his chest in the morning waiting for him to wake. When she thought he was oversleeping she would ever so gently insinuate a careful claw under his left eyelid and raise it – a signal not to be ignored.

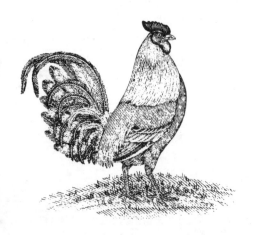